REIKI HEALING

Step-By-Step Guide To Reiki Healing For Beginners

(Reiki Attunement, Reiki Chakras, Reiki Meditation, Reiki Symbols, Reiki Crystals)

Lena Lind & Peter Harris

1

TABLE OF CONTENTS

CHAPTER 1 WHAT IS REIKI?..5

REIKI PRINCIPLES 8

WHAT IS REIKI INITIATION AND HOW CAN IT HELP YOU
....11

THINGS YOU NEED WHEN STARTING YOUR REIKI
PRACTICE 14

**CHAPTER 2 THE IMPORTANCE OF REIKI
ATTUNEMENT** 17

TECHNIQUES FOR REIKI SELF ATTUNEMENT 19

THE HEALING POWER OF REIKI ATTUNEMENTS 23

REIKI HEALING HANDS..26

HEALING POSITIONS FOR REIKI 34

WHAT A REIKI HEALER IS TASKED TO DO 38

BECOME A REIKI MASTER TO ENJOY ALL THE BENEFITS
....41

CHAPTER 3 WHAT ARE REIKI CHAKRAS? 45

THE REIKI ENERGETIC SYSTEM 48

FIVE WAYS TO STRENGTHEN YOUR REIKI ENERGY 52

SELF-HEALING WITH REIKI..58

CHAPTER 4 REIKI CLOTHING..61

CHAPTER 5 HOW TO REIKI? 65

HOW TO LEARN REIKI 69

FOUR FORMS OF REIKI MEDITATION................................72

REIKI MEDITATION TECHNIQUES.......................75

5 WAYS TO USE REIKI................................78

THE BASICS OF REIKI TREATMENT.........................82

USING A PENDULUM DURING REIKI HEALING TREATMENTS 88

CHAPTER 6 SYMBOLS IN REIKI.....................92

HOW TO MAKE REIKI POWER SYMBOLS WORK FOR YOU! 95

CHAPTER 7 REIKI STONES.......................99

ALL ABOUT CRYSTAL HEALING REIKI 103

CHAPTER 1
WHAT IS REIKI?

What is Reiki? Reiki is a Japanese form of Divine healing energy. In different cultures it may be called life force or Chi. Reiki is made up of 2 ancient Japanese kanji characters. The first one means "soul" or "spiritual." Ki, the second kanji symbol means "energy."

Reiki was developed by Master Mikao Usui who was said to have studies Buddhist sutras, martial arts, and other mystical arts. Master Usui fasted for 21 day and saw Reiki energy above his head. He developed Reiki and the symbols from this process and passed on the mysterious knowledge and symbols to several of his students. Some of the Reiki symbols used in healing are from Japanese Buddhism, Shinto and ancient Indian Sanskrit words.

Reiki is not a religion; it is a spiritual healing art that is from the Divine Source. It is used to help the receiver, and the Reiki practitioner heal from the Reiki energy on spiritual, physical, emotional, and mental levels. Reiki can be done at a distance or directly with hands on the receiver. These methods are a catalyst to help one become healed, self-realized, enlightened, and have an open loving heart.

A Reiki practitioner has received attunements from one or more Reiki Masters. These initiations open up and connect the Reiki practitioner to the spiritual healing energy. Anyone can learn this ancient healing art. Anyone can receive this form of healing. It can help heal people, animals, and the earth. It doesn't go against any religion or spiritual practice.

The energy practitioner may lay their hands on the person receiving healing in a set structure of positions from the head, throat, chest, torso, legs and feet. The Reiki practitioner may stray away from these hand positions if they are guided to do so by their intuition or guides. Some Reiki practitioners may have their hands away from your body as well. Reiki may also be done from a distance, even across the globe! These methods can balance the chakras and subtle energy levels.

Practitioners learn the basic hand positions from a Reiki Master in Reiki I. The student then follows with a 21 day cleanse. This process has 12 hand positions that is done for one hour each day. This cleanse connects the new Reiki practitioner daily with this universal energy. It also helps the practitioner become more sensitive to subtle energies in and around their own body.

In Reiki II the student is introduced to the 3 basic, yet powerful symbols which intensify the Reiki energy. In Reiki II, the distance healing symbol is learned. In Reiki III More symbols are introduced. Reiki practitioners may take more classes, but some Masters allow one to teach after 3 classes. If you would like to learn more about Reiki, just ask!

REIKI PRINCIPLES

Reiki is the teaching of the Japanese holistic healing idea. There are a few differences between the Japanese and Western versions although it is really just a difference in the way things are done. One thing is that the Western version doesn't practice breathing techniques. With this practice you sit straight up in a chair and breathe in and out through the nose. At that time the energy enters through the top of the head.

Another difference between the two is the ways of treatment. In traditional Japanese healing people go to meetings every week and meditation work is done on separate parts, and with Western areas, the healing is usually done on the whole body. Also in Western areas there are three degrees or levels.

The first Reiki Degree course can be varied depending on the teacher. Some teachers have two classes over a two day period. Other teachers have four sessions spread over an extended period. Students are taught meditation and hand placement for healing. At that time they can heal themselves and others.

In the second degree level students learn the use of symbols to enhance the connection between the healer and recipient. The use of these symbols helps to do the healing over distance and time. You can heal people without being with them. In Japan it has been known to take ten to twenty years to attain the second degree. It is dependent on the teacher.

In Reiki, there is always learning involved. As with the third degree, there is a time that it takes to study and practice. It depends on the teacher as to how long it takes to attain third degree status. It could be a day or a year or more. When you are obtaining the third degree you are given another symbol.

It is thought that Reiki healing is used on the front and back of the body equally. It is usually started at the head and neck and then the other parts of the body. Reiki does not use medicine or instruments but feeling, blowing, tapping, and massaging. It is a practice that uses the energies that surround all of us always.

Many Western practitioners usually use a standard twelve positions for whole body healing. The recipient is asked to lay down when this is being done. The hands are usually held at each position for five minutes. Some people say that they get a warm feeling where the treatment is being applied. This is also a hand off treatment as the hands are held as few centimeters away from the recipient.

There is really no governing board for Reiki practitioners but there are organizations that want to standardize Reiki practices. If that should happen the practice might be under government regulation and that could be a fatal blow the practitioners of today and of the future.

WHAT IS REIKI INITIATION AND HOW CAN IT HELP YOU

Reiki, as is well-known, is a derivation of Buddhist philosophies, which a Buddhist monk name Masai Ukui derived in Japan during a spiritual retreat in the 19th century. Reiki has become massively popular in Western culture due to the claims made on its behalf - it is stated by reiki teachers and master that reiki can help ease a sufferer's pain while supplementing his or her regular medical treatment.

This is something to remember: reiki is not a replacement for mainstream modern medicine. Buddhist philosophy explicitly states that it is designed for the easing of a person's pain, and reiki itself is derived from such teachings. Reiki works on spiritual energies, which are contained in the body of the sufferer and, if mis-aligned, cause pain. These energy or 'ki' sites are the basis of reiki practice, and there are three levels of proficiency. Let's take a quick look at each.

During a reiki course the student undergoes a process of attunement, or initiation, under the tutelage of a Reiki master.

Very simply, this allows the student to use and receive more of the universal spiritual energy circulating around us. The rate at which this energy spins differs, and so there must be different techniques and methods of dealing with it.

These methods are taught at the ascending levels of reiki studenthood, at the final stage of which one is considered a reiki master. These levels are Reiki 1, Reiki 2, and the third, Level 3, at which one is considered a master and can go forth and train more budding recruits into the ranks of the reiki elite. It is possible, with the recent advances made in the teaching of reiki, to advance to the second level in a matter of mere days.

The attunement process starts with the master reflecting this universal energy, via his or her hands, into the body of the sufferer. The person's body is then searched for hidden blockages of the energy, the 'ki', which is the basis of every human being's spiritual self.

In order, the process goes through the following three stages:

The Reiki initiation level 1 works by stimulating the body to receive a small amount of spiritual energy, and to prepare it to receive more. This is a complete novice level. It also makes the person who receives this initiation capable of retaining that attunement for the rest of his or her life. The basic hand positions of reiki, as well as some of its history, are taught, and at the end of each experience - always relaxing and spiritually good for both master and student - the student can progress to the second level, or choose to remain at level 1 and continue to experience the good it does to him or her.

The Reiki initiation level 2 involves the teaching of certain symbols, e.g. the mental symbol, which then allow the student to prepare for the third level, which is where the student achieves mastery.

THINGS YOU NEED WHEN STARTING YOUR REIKI PRACTICE

Are you a trained in Reiki and want to start making a living of it? Are you setting up your own Reiki practice? Congratulations! You are going to make a difference in many people's lives. So what do you need when starting out, apart from the legalities and a location to practice? In this article I will go through the equipment that you will need and I hope it will prove useful information.

1. Reiki Table. This can mean an important investment as some of them don't come very cheap. But don't just look at the price. You need to see the whole picture. A high quality table, with a long warranty, will pay you its cost many times over. You need to make sure the measures are adequate and that it is portable. Make sure it is sturdy and that it feels stable. Your clients won't feel secure when lying down otherwise. The Reiki tables differ from normal massage tables in one aspect. Reiki tables have room for your legs so that you can sit next to it comfortably. Massage tables usually don't have this feature because the therapist spends more time standing then sitting down.

2. Reiki Table Carrying case. Some sellers will include a carrying case in the package, and if not I very much recommend getting one separately. Maybe you have clients that are too ill to get to your practice and you need to do a lot of home visits. This can easily be arranged if your equipment is light and portable. A carrying case can be useful even if you don't move about a lot, when storing it for example.

3. Reiki Table accessories. This is up to every Reiki practitioner but the basics are usually face and head rest, adjustable arm rest and bolster.

4. Clean linens, preferably white. There are special ones made for massage and Reiki tables that fit perfectly.

5. Blankets and pillows to assure maximum comfort.
Choose natural materials such as cotton, not synthetics.

6. Decoration. This is very subjective. Some Reiki practitioners will decorate the room with crystals, posters, candles. This is really up to each and every one of us but make sure you choose only authentic products. You should feel a positive energy when walking into the practice, and so should your clients.

7. Relaxing music and stereo equipment.

8. Crystals. Some Reiki experts say that crystals used during Reiki will help the healing and energy balancing. And they also speed up the recovery process. You can start with a small collection of stones. They shouldn't be too heavy nor too small that you'll lose them. Flat stones will stay on the spot more easily. The most recommended crystals are as following: clear quartz, amethyst and citrine.

CHAPTER 2
THE IMPORTANCE OF REIKI ATTUNEMENT

In the magical world of Reiki, everything is said to be possible. One is not only able to heal one's self, whether one is ill physically, mentally, or emotionally, one is also able to remove from a sick loved one the pain and hurt that diseases of the mind and those physical in nature bring through a proper execution of reiki therapy.

What more, you can actually execute the attunement that comes with the therapy long distance. Therefore, even if the sick loved one is in a hospital bed miles from where you are, you can still hear your loved one. You can perform the reiki attunement process in the comforts of your home and provided you did executed properly, it'll surely work.

Now, you can joyously say goodbye to long distance travels, hello reiki therapy! Say adieu too to horrific hospital bills that loved ones wants you to shoulder, hello fast recovery and good health!

This is the power that reiki practitioners have been bestowed with through the process of attunement. Reiki, by the way, is a Japanese healing art form that came from the root words "Rei", which means "Higher Power", and "Ki" that is translated to mean "life force energy".

An ancient healing technique that had its beginnings in the South Pacific island of Japan hundreds of years ago, it has today transformed itself to become an alternative form of medication or treatment for many well-known illnesses such as cancer, severe migraines, and many others.

To the fascinated Westerners, reiki therapy, the practice of which actually, has become a lifestyle choice believing that with regular attunement sessions on one's body, and possibly on other people's bodies as well, one becomes more balanced emotionally and mentally. This, in turn, should result to healthier food choices and an affinity for physical activities.

It is because of these wonderful benefits that regular attunement sessions should be done. Attunements are important in Reiki because it is how a Reiki Master is able to release "Ki" from his spirit and share it with a Reiki Practitioner. Attunement is sometimes referred to in Reiki as a ceremony of the spirit, as it is from one's spirit that the "life force energy" flows and is transferred to those who need healing.

This is how a reiki therapy takes place. This is how healing happens. This is why so many people are fascinated with Reiki and after one attunement session have become avid fans and practitioners of the Japanese healing art form. Attunement kicks it all off and from there comes healing.

TECHNIQUES FOR REIKI SELF ATTUNEMENT

Reiki is natural healing with energy. Reiki heals by bringing in balance and harmony to those who embrace it. Everything and anything in this world is made up of different energy that vibrates at different frequencies. Because energy cannot be destroyed, it remains in its constant state until it is converted.

Free techniques for Reiki self-attunement allow one to replace negative energy with positive energy in order heal the mind, body, and soul.

Listed below are the 4 free techniques on how to self-attune yourself to Reiki to better understand how simple and effective this energy healing can be.

1. Preparation to self-attune yourself to Reiki is important. Meditation starting one week prior to your self-attunement session is best. Meditation helps clear and relax the mind and body. It allows us to open up on a more spiritual level. One should also stop smoking and drinking alcohol one day prior to self-attunement since these can cause blockage in the body.

2. On the day of self-attunement, it is helpful to sit in a meditative position. Try and imagine all negative energies releasing from your body through your crown chakra. Your crown chakra is located at the top of your head. When I do this, sometimes I imagine an angel coming down with a

bucket to collect my negative thoughts and energies and rid them from me. (Picturing an action like the angel works best for me.)

3. Mentally repeat to yourself which Reiki level you wish to be attuned. If you wish to start with Reiki Level 1, then repeat this to yourself and meditate on it.

4. Feel the Reiki level that you request enter through your crown chakra and flowing through each and every part of your body. It helps to picture this Reiki level as a white light. Enjoy the meditative feeling you are in for roughly 30 - 45 minutes. Once your whole body clears, you can ground yourself.

There are a lot more different techniques to Reiki self-attunement. The above provides a brief lesson for someone interested in self-attuning them self to Reiki. A person who embraces these techniques to heal themselves, will think clearer, and find that they have more energy to perform in their daily lives.

THE HEALING POWER OF REIKI ATTUNEMENTS

There is possibly no treatment to physical ailment as impressive healing achieved by free Reiki attunements. Reiki is a practice of healing with the power of a spiritual light derived from the power of love and serenity. Achieved power to heal by means of meditation and practice is a controversial topic that is winning the opinion among Western practitioners of health.

While there is not yet concrete scientific data that attunements achieved through Reiki enlightenment hold credibility in improving a patient's state of health; there is overwhelming evidence from believers who say the power of Reiki has performed miracles in their lives.

Since the time of its inception over five thousand years ago, Reiki has been believed to be a highly coveted ability to heal. Reiki attunements are said to be responsible for hundreds - if not thousands - of otherwise inexplicable cases of astonishing and virtually instantaneous eradication of an ailments. Those who have experienced Reiki healing have adopted a firm belief in the power of holistic healing.

Reiki is widely believed to require a high level of consciousness to spirituality and an ability to comprehend that which - in words - may not have a description. Reiki symbolism can only be roughly translated. Like the language in which it was born, Sanskrit, there are hardly words adequate enough to truly capture the essence of what is expressed in the characters. There is a deep understanding of the flow of our life force, and its relationship to the Universe in which we are encompassed.

Reiki is a very deep, philosophical belief system, whose execution is divided into many tiers. Levels of free Reiki attunements to the human body are limitless. There are Reiki 'prescriptions' to multiple emotional disturbances. These types of ailments, including Schizophrenia and other psychotic disorders; are thought in some roots of Reiki to be caused by influencing factors from previous lives. That is, however, contingent upon the fact that it was an illness with which the afflicted was born.

Emotional disturbances that may occur later in life are attributed to a sick spirits conflicted reaction to the heartache that is caused by earthly greed and sin. These types of self-inflicted ailments of the mind are healed differently than those caused by anguish carried over from past lives.

In addition to Reiki taking responsibility for some of the most extreme cases of mental illness, there have also been world-wide occurrences of various physical deficiencies having been reversed. There are a wide variety of sources that provide detailed attunement techniques inspired by Reiki used to cure tooth aches, cold symptoms, and other natural causes of pain.

Reiki has been used for centuries as one of the most profound healing methods ever known to man. For the great many who scoff, there are an equal amount of believers. Among the believers are real life people who have experienced the power of Reiki.

You can investigate yourself online, to see if you agree with any of the principle ideals that outline the fundamental quantum physics that have made millions of believers of the power of free Reiki attunements.

REIKI HEALING HANDS

Healing hands could be the term offered to persons that have been attuned to the healing power of Reiki Healing and can perform Reiki channeling of this power by way of their hands.

What is Reiki?

Reiki is usually a kind of hands on healing, with its origins in India plus the East dating back a lot of thousands of years to the time ahead of Christ and Buddha. Usui Reiki is a strategy of reiki developed by Dr Mikao Usui in the 19th century. Usui himself produced the name REIKI, Rei which means Universal and Ki meaning Life force.

Usui created this system of reiki to ensure that any person could practice hands on healing. He wanted reiki to become universal so that whatever religious or cultural backgrounds you held you'd have the ability to turn out to be a reiki master. Adults and kids alike can practice Usui Reiki.

Reiki may be the gift of vitality and self-preservation encoded into the genetic makeup of all God's creatures. It's the higher self's connection to the universal power that breathes life into all living tissues. We are all born with the omniscient wisdom to heal and preserve life, with all living things connected by the Universal Life Force, the nonphysical ubiquitous energy that provides life to just about every living organism.

How are you able to Obtain Reiki?

It is possible to obtain Reiki from a certified Reiki practitioner. You are able to also perform Reiki on oneself by understanding Reiki. We think that The Essence Of Reiki home Study Course would be the greatest home study course about, to find out about Reiki, we employed this course and discovered it very uncomplicated to follow and enjoyable. Right after completing the course you may be a certified Usui Reiki Master and Animal Reiki Master.

The Benefits of Hands on Reiki Healing

Reiki can help you boost every single aspect of your life and support to retain ongoing wellness and prevent illness. It is actually for everybody and can be applied to heal adults, youngsters, babies, an unborn youngster and also pets. It's a safe and straightforward therapy option that can be made use of to complement and enhance the effects with the regular wellness care an individual receives within the hospital or wellness center.

Indeed, Reiki is made use of within a broad range of settings like hospitals, hospices, cancer support groups, post-operative recovery as well as in drug rehabilitation. Reiki can also be applied with other natural healing therapies which include meditation, crystals and aroma therapy, with Reiki reinforcing the effect of these healing therapies.

Our Knowledge of Healing Hands

As Usui Reiki Masters we've received and performed Reiki on numerous occasions. We really feel that the healing power of Reiki is an extraordinary thing and we really feel extremely relaxed afterwards. The most beneficial approach to fully grasp what healing hands are or really feel like would be to experience it for your self Reiki Hand Positions.

As soon as you've received the very first degree attunement, from a Reiki Master that you are ready to work using the universal life force. Nevertheless, it really is vital that you just realize as with every profession there's a must 1st practice and master the abilities connected with healing including the correct Reiki Hand Positions to get a Reiki Self Therapy. Madam Takata taught her students to heal themselves initially, then their families, then their good friends. Only then did she think they would be adequately qualified and in a position to operate as a practitioner and heal other people.

Finding out the Reiki Hand Positions can be comparable to when someone very first learns to drive an auto they need time, practice and experience to master what appears to be a rather complicated set of procedures. Nevertheless, within a fairly brief space of time they're able to drive safely and effortlessly as they unconsciously manage the car and all the many abilities associated with driving.

Likewise with time, practice and experience you might master the skills and strategies associated with art of Reiki healing such as the Reiki Hand Positions. Treat the early months as a finding out encounter, just about like an apprenticeship; this can provide you with the time you'll want to develop your self-confidence and expertise. Keep in mind the more you operate with Reiki then a lot more intuitive you are going to become, your energy vibration will likely be raised and you'll develop and expertise a new joyful consistency inside your life.

Making use of the Reiki Hand Positions when performing a reiki self-healing could be the starting point for individual development and self-discovery. Reiki will not be just a tool for healing; it also brings protection, prevention and private transformation on all levels.

As you progress along your new path, inevitably you are going to come up against obstacles and setbacks in your life that typically appear like the whole ocean front, but with Reiki you'll have the strength to cope with them as though they may be but pebbles on the beach. Even when you under no circumstances use Reiki to heal anyone but yourself, you can discover a brand new sense of balance and peace in your life.

There's no other process of self-treatment as simple and as useful as Reiki. Simply because Reiki is usually accessible to you, whenever you really feel tired, stressed, have any aches or pains, it is possible to alleviate them by merely laying your hands on your body. The infinite wisdom of Reiki will go to wherever it can be essential.

Recharge your batteries every day, not just when issues, difficulties, anxiousness or illnesses arise. Day-to-day self-remedy will support to prevent sickness and disease, and bring your life into focus and balance speedily. Every time you use Reiki on yourself, you raise your self-esteem and self-adore. You'll discover your mission in life and develop it into additional compassion and love.

Instead of receiving stress in the normal actions you make contact with each day such as traffic jams; meetings, interviews, going to the physicians or dentist, waiting in queues, your youngsters requires and your family responsibilities to name but a few, enable Reiki into your life and let Reiki develop into a brand new way of life to you.

Reiki is actually a gift to be savored and enjoyed. Keep in mind the more you use Reiki the stronger and much more profound it becomes. Every day use could extend your personal life by quite a few years.

You can find a number of positive aspects to become gained, which take place with no any effort from an everyday Reiki self-treatment like:

- Reiki will unwind you if you are stressed
- Reiki brings about deep relaxation
- Reiki centers your thoughts if you are confused
- Reiki energizes you if you feel drained
- Reiki calms you after you are frightened
- Reiki focuses your thoughts and helps you to resolve issues
- Reiki relieves pain
- Reiki accelerates natural healing of wounds
- Reiki improves wellness
- Reiki gradually clears up chronic troubles
- Reiki assists prevents the improvement of disease
- Reiki detoxifies the body
- Reiki dissolves energy blockages

- Reiki releases emotional wounds

- Reiki increases the vibrational frequency in the physique

- Reiki assists transform unfavorable yourself with Reiki

There is certainly no right or wrong approach to work with Reiki on oneself. As you become much more experienced with all the Reiki energy you can intuitively move your hands to wherever it feels right. Having said that, should you be aware of a specific problem which includes an injury or pain, then you should place your hands directly over that area to begin with, and follow up with a full self-treatment.

In the beginning, it is often very best to follow a set procedure using the chakra points.

Once you have mastered the hand positions you can then leave each and every self-treatment up to your own intuition. You may wish to function with music to add the right relaxing mood. Discover a place where you won't be disturbed if possible. Normally you would spend three to five minutes on every position.

Even so, time is typically short, but recall a little Reiki is better than no Reiki. On completion in the self-therapy drink a large glass of purified water. Close your eyes and go inside and pay attention for the thoughts and emotions that have arisen during the session. You may really feel light headed, and for those who must rest, or sit down to get a brief time, allow yourself this time.

If you feel you must continue to function on a specific area with the physique, even if you've got completed a full self-therapy employing the reiki hand positions, then go with your intuition; often listen to your thoughts and body. Remember the reiki healing hand positions are only a guide? Use your intuition.

HEALING POSITIONS FOR REIKI

Teaching Reiki is much easier when students have a lot of questions. Here are the most common questions that come up in our classes: Do I sit or stand when giving Reiki? How long do I stay at each position? How long does a Reiki session take? What do I do after I've completed all the healing positions?

Healing Positions while giving Reiki

Sit or stand so you are stable and can hold a position comfortably for 5 to 10 minutes. Some teachers suggest beginning a healing at the head while others suggest beginning at the feet. Experiment to determine what feels right for each person you heal. Trust your intuition in each situation. Be mindful and honor any thoughts, feelings or instructions that arise during healing. Reiki always goes where it is needed, so relax and let it flow.

The photo in my author profile shows suitable positions for placing your hands during a healing. For a larger and clearer image of the chakra system, visit my webpage following the link at the bottom of this page

Apply Reiki directly to the seven major chakras, plus knees and feet. As you gain experience and knowledge, you will intuitively know the best location to place your hands. Initially, let your hands hover 25 centimeters (12 inches)

above the body and gradually get closer. Decide if you will make physical contact at each chakra or stay in the aura a short distance away. At most chakras, you can touch a person's body directly. At private or sensitive areas such as the throat, breasts and genitals, maintain a distance of about 10 centimeters (4 inches). Use common sense along with mutual respect and Reiki will flow optimally. Some healers give Reiki only on the front of the body while others give it both front and back. Trust your intuition to decide where to apply your hands, depending on the time available, symptoms and the setting where you perform the healing.

Duration of Healing

Observe the flow of Reiki in your hands. You may feel warmth, tingling, tickling, pulsing, coolness or maybe nothing at all. When the sensations change, this indicates that you can proceed to the next position. If in doubt, remain at each position about 5 minutes. The brow and crown chakras may require more energy and time.

Overall, a healing session may take 45 to 90 minutes, depending on the depth of the healing that you intend. For example, if you are at home with your brother who is feeling very stressed and has a sore back, a 90 minute Reiki session covering front and back may be suitable. With children, 1 or 2 minutes per chakra is sufficient; a complete session may require only 10 minutes.

Some people may not be skeptical but they simply don't know what you're talking about when you mention Reiki to help them with their pain. In cases like these, keep your healing process very simple.

If somebody has pain in one specific area, use Reiki directly on that location. If for example you are sitting in the library with a friend who has a headache, applying Reiki at just one or two head positions is sufficient. This should be followed up with a more thorough healing session when you get to a more suitable location.

WHAT A REIKI HEALER IS TASKED TO DO

Reiki as a healing technique does not only give one the privilege to become a Reiki healer but at the same time puts on the shoulders of the healer certain responsibilities by which he is trained to live up to. It is not as simply as getting a "know" on the healing technique and use it whenever you just feel like it like it is just a passing fad or hobby.

The healers of Reiki could have quite vast and varied tasks at hand. Perhaps the most basic among these responsibilities would have to be always being in tune with the divine power of chi or ki. This is where the power to heal and bless comes from. How does a Reiki healer do this? He has to spend sufficient time in prayer or meditation every day.

This should enable him to access this energy source and at the same time be able to use it for other people to benefit from. The truth about the healing power of a Reiki master or practitioner depends on the time that he spends in prayer and meditation by which enhances the energy source and making it potentially ready for sharing and beneficial healing of others.

Note that as healers of Reiki are able to keep up with this task, so are they tasked to do the very same thing for themselves - to be empowered and in tune at all times for them to heal their own selves.

As the healer, you are blessed with the potential to be well at all times and at the same time have more access to the plan and order of the divine beings and powers. And this said, as a healer or Reiki to be in such a position would have to be a tremendous blessing.

As a Reiki healer, you are also expected to keep your temporal body clean - which means free from toxic substances. The reason or this is that this enables their physical health and constitution to become conducive to the energy flow that is powerful and whereby functions through their own hands.

The healer knows that the body is the living vessel by which you are tasked to keep clean at all times. Would you rather make your medium of healing by which others benefit from rather dirty and intoxicated? The medium should be at all times kept pure. This means that you should be careful even with the quality of food that you are ingesting.

Finally, there should be an adherence to the fact that the divine power and energy should at all times be never used for self-interest.

The healer is but a steward to this magnificent power, hence he should never take it to be his own and him being the true reason of healing. A true Reiki healer understands that he is the caretaker of this divine power and not the possessor of it!

BECOME A REIKI MASTER TO ENJOY ALL THE BENEFITS

What is Reiki? This energy healing art allows people to overcome certain health issues and achieve high levels of stress management. To learn Reiki or become a Reiki Master is to introduce yourself to a wonderful form of self-realization and to allow you to achieve great emotional balance in your life and for the lives of those around you.

Many people learn Reiki and become a Reiki Master purely for the benefits which they realize for themselves. Reiki healing has been around for centuries, with the Western variety emerging in the early 1900s.

This healing art is quickly being accepted into mainstream medicine after years of being viewed as alternative!

To learn Reiki is not difficult. The most important prerequisite is an openness to explore the healing arty and energy healing. Complete training involves three levels, which progress to the Master / Teacher level.

A brief description of the three stages is included below:

First Degree

At this level, the student learns the workings of Reiki. The student also discovers the various types of Reiki which are practiced. There is also an initiation, or Reiki attunement, to the first level. This will be the student's first experience of Reiki energy from the learn Reiki perspective.

The sensations are very different to those experienced during a Reiki healing session and must be enjoyed to be believed. The attunement received at the first level shows the student how to balance energy and use it for procedures such as stress management. Even a first level attunement is very beneficial all on its own.

The attunement can be in person or remote. The only important variable is the experience and pedigree of the Master. This is why some of the Reiki course online has become incredibly popular, because those led by experienced Reiki Masters are among the best ways to learn Reiki.

Second Degree

The second level expands on the first level and introduces the concept of distance healing. Because the energy used for healing is the energy of the patient the Master does not need to be present to successfully treat the patient. The same is very true for those who learn Reiki! You don't need the Master to be present. You just need access to the Master and a willingness to embrace the concept!

The energy vibration at second level is entirely different to the first level. The first level can be said to deal with primarily the physical level whereas the second level also introduces emotional, spiritual, and mental healing.

Third Degree

This is the pinnacle for those who set out to learn Reiki. Only the third degree gives you exposure to all of the Reiki symbols and their correct use and application. Students also complete their crystal healing training and learn how the different energy sources and flows operate. Upon completion of the third level you have become a Reiki Master and can train others. You can also perform all of the Reiki attunements.

CHAPTER 3
WHAT ARE REIKI CHAKRAS?

The different Reiki chakras are used in the practice of Reiki in order to bring focus and universal energy directly to the healer. Its purpose is to absorb all possible cosmic energy and distribute it evenly upon the body of the healer.

Clearing the different Reiki chakras is a good way to start the whole Reiki healing process. As the Reiki energy increases, the life processes from the earth to the spiritual world progresses as well, leading to a step in complete human growth. But clearing the chakras used in Reiki is dangerous if done without the proper guidance and proper supervision - if one is not fully ready to receive the chakras, a surge of energy can be overwhelming and harmful. It can lead to a possible disorientation, depravity, physical pain, and even mental breakdown.

The first Reiki Chakra is located at the base of the spine area. It helps in the body's survival, security, safety and the ability to be grounded to the earthly plane. Its physical functions are responsible for the excretion and digestion. It is responsible for the proper functioning of the small intestine and the colon, as well the sex glands, the hips, the legs, the lower back, and the rectum.

The second Reiki Chakra is found just above the genitals. It covers the individual's sexuality, self-esteem, personal power and the need to control one's emotions. It has physical influence on the ovaries, the fallopian tubes, the pelvic area, the lumbar spine, the kidneys, the bladder and the large intestines. It is also considered as the center for the body's cleansing, purification, and total health. If not attended to, it can have serious effects on the adrenal glands, leading to ulcer. It can also cause other nervous disorders and chronic fatigue.

The third Chakra is located two fingers just above the naval. When it is opened, it allows a person to function normally even when the person feels distressed. It provides the person the capability to connect, have long term relationships and can even influence into having a loving family and a happy home.

If it is abused, it can have profound effects on the sympathetic nervous system, muscular energy, heartbeat, digestion and circulation. If this chakra is blocked, the energy moving from past diaphragm will be hindered thus the energy cannot be transmitted to other parts of the body.

The fourth Chakra is located at the eight cervical vertebra of the spine opposite the heart. It allows one to sympathize with the vibrations of other astral entities so that one can instinctively understand the greater energies and atmospheres. This fourth chakra has physical influence on the thymus (located at the center of the chest behind the upper breast bone). The thymus is responsible for the proper utilization of the amino competence factor, that helps create the body's immunity to disease.

THE REIKI ENERGETIC SYSTEM

But what energetic system are the principles of a Reiki practice based on? As Reiki is a Japanese practice that was created in the early 1900s we are aware that (as with many martial arts and Ki practices that were formalized in Japan at the same time - karate, judo, aikido) the hara or tanden were considered to be the center of the body's energetic powerhouse.

The word hara literally means stomach, abdomen or belly in Japanese. Energy is stored in this point of the body from where it expands throughout the whole body.

Usui Mikao's teachings focus on building the energy in the hara. From Hawayo Takata's diary notes it can be seen that she too was taught to practice in this manner. Once the system of Reiki became more westernized in the 1980s the chakra system (an energetic system from India that has been incorporated into the New Age movement) was introduced and replaced this system - the chakra system is now commonly used in the West

In traditional Japanese teachings and exercises today the hara system is still the main focus for building a person's energy. There are, in fact, two other energy centers in the body according to the Japanese energetic system. One is the head and the other is the heart. In the Japanese Art of Reiki we have called these the Three Diamonds. By linking all three areas the practitioner creates unity and balance. Most important, however, is to first develop the lower hara, as this is the body's central axis point.

Re-establishing this connection with the Original Energy through the hara will ensure good health and recovery from illness. There is always access to a reliable source of strength whenever needed.

An inner attitude results from first focusing on the hara. From this central point there is an ability to cope with everyday tasks and sudden emergencies with an ease of understanding. This allows appropriate action to be taken in a balanced and unprejudiced manner.

1. Lower hara (approximately 3 inches (8cms) below the naval)

In this center, Original Energy is stored. This is the energy you are born with, the energy that is the essence of your life and gives you your life's purpose. The Original Energy is not only the energy you receive from your parents when you are conceived but most importantly it is the energetic connection between you and the universal life force. When the singular term hara is mentioned it is the lower hara that is being discussed. This is the symbolic energetic center for Earth Ki.

2. Middle hara (at the heart centre)

The energy in this centre is connected with emotions. It is 'human' energy connected with human experience. Through this centre you learn your life's process. From childhood through to adulthood and back to being a child. When you are a child you are without experience and as you grow older you become a child with experience. This is the symbolic energetic centre for Heart Ki.

3. Upper hara (third eye area).

This is the energy connected with your spirit. When you are connected with this centre you may see colors or you might have psychic ability. It is important for you not to become unbalanced and keep yourself centered. If you can use this energy in a balanced way, you can see beyond the immediate. This is the symbolic energetic centre for Heaven Ki.

The three diamonds of Earth Ki, Heaven Ki and Heart Ki are at the foundation of the system of Reiki. They are also at the crux of many facets of Japanese culture, religion and philosophy.

A diamond is often used as an analogy of the self in Buddhism. Each and every day a practitioner polishes the diamond by performing his or her practice. This is a constant task for humans who, in this earthly realm, attract dirt: becoming muddy and tarnished. A diamond is so sharp that it can cut through almost anything humanity attaches itself to, bringing back the true essence of life as seen in the perfection of a sparkling diamond.

FIVE WAYS TO STRENGTHEN YOUR REIKI ENERGY

TECHNIQUE 1: DRY BATHING (KENYOKU HO)

Although this is by far the most complex energy 'trick' of the five, it is still relatively simple. Doing it before each Reiki session will definitely make a difference to the flow of energy.

Method:

- Put your right hand on your left shoulder, breathe into your hara (i.e. the 2nd chakra - located about 5cm below your belly button), and sweep diagonally - exhaling forcefully - across the front of your body down to your right hip.

- (By 'sweep', we mean brushing your hand over your body as if you were 'sweeping' dust away from your shoulder, past your hip and onto the ground.)

- Put your left hand on your right shoulder, inhale into your hara, and 'sweep' - exhaling - down to your left hip.

- Put your hand back on your left shoulder, inhale, and sweep your hand - exhaling - down to your right hip.

- Extend your left arm out in front of your body, palm facing upwards, arm horizontal to the ground. Put your right hand on your left shoulder - inhale into your hara - and 'sweep' along your arm - exhaling - all the way past the left fingertips.

- Repeat the process on your opposite side by extending your right hand palm facing upwards in front of your body (arm horizontal to the ground), placing your left hand on your right shoulder, inhaling into your hara, and sweeping along your right arm - exhaling - all the way past the right fingertips.

- Extend your left arm out in front of your body, palm facing upwards, arm horizontal to the ground. Put your right hand on your left shoulder - inhale into your hara - and 'sweep' along your arm - exhaling - all the way past the left fingertips.

- Let your arms hang down by the sides of your body and feel any energetic currents that may arise (most probably in your arms and hands).

- Gassho (join your hands together in prayer position [namaste] in front of your chest) and give thanks.

TECHNIQUE 2: RUBBING HANDS TOGETHER

Rub your hands together vigorously for ten seconds before giving yourself or another Reiki. This will stimulate the energetic channels in your hand, thus making it easier for the Reiki energy to flow.

TECHNIQUE 3: KEEP FINGERS TOGETHER AND HANDS CUPPED

Reiki will generally flow more strongly if you keep your fingers together (although the thumb may, at times, separate from the other fingers).

Mrs Takata, the founder of Western Reiki, apparently proclaimed: 'Scattered hands, scattered energy'. She was right, although you should naturally never be dogmatic (sometimes, after all, you may in fact desire a more spread out sort of energy).

That said, 9 times out of 10 you will feel more if you keep your fingers together.

The same can also be said for keeping your hands held cupped rather than flat on the body. The reasons for this are not exactly clear, but try it if you are not already doing so. The energy almost always seems to flow better.

TECHINQUE 4: Hover above Each Hand Position before Touching the Body

A good way to get a stronger connection to each Reiki position is to hover above it with your hands before lowering them onto the body.

The trick is to wait until you get an energetic connection and only then put your hands on the body. For some reason this makes it easier to connect to the Reiki energy of each position.

TECHNIQUE 5: Keep One Hand on the Body When Changing Hand Positions

To keep the energetic connection going (and build momentum, thus strengthening it), it is a good idea not to take both hands off your body when changing positions (the same applies when you give Reiki to someone else).

Keep one hand grounded while you move the other. Then anchor the one you have moved, and move the one you had kept grounded. That way the energetic space and connection you have established is not short-circuited.

SELF-HEALING WITH REIKI

Reiki can be used to heal others. But more importantly, it can very well be used to heal your own self. There are many ways you can do so.

Every one of us has unique personal qualities. And these qualities can be improved greatly to make you a better person. You can turn these qualities into abilities and skills, which could help you greatly in life. However, we must live well and wisely. That's the only way you can lead a life of development, growth, and healing.

Try to look back in your life. How many choices have you made that turned your life around? Every decision that you do has a powerful effect to your own existence. Your decisions become a part of what you are and who you become. Not all your choices are correct. It is but human nature to make mistakes. But what's more important is for you to learn from your errors. If you are able to understand your wrongness, you are not likely to repeat the blunder.

If you are in a spot wherein your life is in a tumble because of your wrong decisions in life, Reiki can outwardly help you to correct it. Try to heal, change, and recreate your life towards the correct path. Reiki's self-healing techniques can be very beneficial for this purpose.

One good teaching of Reiki revolves around balance. Know that the whole universe exists in a balanced state. As such, all your life's difficulties have solutions. There can't be a problem without a solution. Every challenging situation has a way out. This is what the concept of universal balance implies.

In order to find the solution, it is very important that you have the definiteness of purpose. Sustain your will and purpose. Over time, good things will happen to you. Having a definite purpose always produces the best results. Set your goals and purposes early on. Then focus on it up until you are able to attain it. Use Reiki to your advantage to further your purpose. In time, self-healing will be attained. If you pursue your purpose with passion, you will be healed faster.

Keep in mind that the mind acts similar to a magnet. It attracts everything that you think of. Think hard about your goal. And the attraction would compound greatly. Set your mind towards your objectives. This is very helpful in improving yourself or any of your qualities. Hold the thought, believe in it definitely, and know that it will happen. Sooner or later, it will. The power of Reiki is based on this fact.

Remember that everyone has their own purpose in life. Therefore, everybody has a task to accomplish. And those tasks may require one or more special abilities. This is why you need to heal and improve yourself so that your personal qualities will be honed to perfection. It is part of your task to fully express your talents to the whole world. The Divine Being gave these talents to you. You are supposed to use them for everybody's benefits.

CHAPTER 4
REIKI CLOTHING

Is it possible to acquire the benefits of Reiki without actually practicing it? Is there any other way the energy of Reiki can be communicated? Is there a way to effectively channel the energy of Reiki to others?

Many Reiki healers were involved in various experiments to see if it was possible to impart the healing power others by different means. Thanks to those millions of experiments, now we know various ways in which Reiki can be channeled to others. The most popular way in which energy can be obtained is from Reiki infused clothing.

What is Reiki Clothing?

Reiki clothing refers to clothing that is wholly infused with Reiki energy by an efficient Reiki healer. After a short meditation session, the clothes are infused with Reiki energy. This attire imparts the Reiki energy to those who wear it and surrounds the person with the power of Reiki. Wearing Reiki clothing has a good deal of benefits and you will feel the impact of the Reiki clothing when you switch back to your regular outfit. That is when you will realize the immense transition you went through in all three dimensions of your life - your mind, body and soul.

When can Reiki Clothing be worn?

Reiki clothing holding such great energy can be worn anytime of the day. It can be worn through the day when you are most active going about your daily chores; this way you will be able to carry out your tasks with ease and without your energy being drained. You can also wear this clothing when you go to bed.

This is the time when your body is in recharge mode and if you wear Reiki clothes while sleeping, it will greatly assist the rejuvenation process. You can wear it during celebrations or gatherings to add more radiance to yourself. Reiki clothes are also ideal to wear during any religious ceremonies; the energy would help you connect deep with the superior being.

What materials can be used to make Reiki Clothes?

Reiki clothes are made using different types of cloth, but what really matters is the energy charged into the clothing. Reiki clothing is made from cotton, Lycra, cashmere, silk etc. Other clothes includes tee shirts, denim jackets, tunics, skirts, pants, tank tops and almost all other fashionable forms of clothing. Reiki clothes made from silk are quite popular as it is believed that the properties of silk greatly complement Reiki.

Benefits of Reiki Clothing:

Wearing Reiki clothes has numerous benefits:

1. Balances your body vibrations and revitalizing you from within.

2. Let's you receive enjoy all the benefits of Reiki energy.

3. Helps your body to heal itself.

4. Increases your spirit and energy, and also keeps your energy levels from becoming exhausted.

5. Boosts your confidence and enhances your way of life.

CHAPTER 5
HOW TO REIKI?

THE WONDER OF REIKI

Reiki is a Japanese word for describing Universal life force energy. Reiki is also known as Chi and Prana. This is the same energy which makes the plants grow, the tides flow, and the wind blow. In fact it is everywhere and in everything in the Universe.

Many stories abound about its re-discovery have been handed down orally through the ages, and as with any good story various changes creep in depending on the ear that hears it! The common accepted facts are that it was rediscovered by Dr Mikao Usui towards the end of the 19th century, during a deep state of meditation. During this meditation he was able to see various symbols and instinctively understood ways to harness this universal energy to heal one's own body. After his life-transforming experience and discovery of universal healing energy he put his new found skills to good use during the violent earthquake in Japan (1923) and reportedly helped many people back to health.

Initially Dr Usui simply healed people in individual sessions through the amazing power of reiki but eventually it was taught to students. This has resulted in Reiki being widely available in every part of the world today. However, it is imperative that you pick a qualified and adept teacher if you wish to learn or receive Reiki.

Reiki works on 4 levels to support holistic healing in the individual:

- Physical - It alleviates pain, detoxifies the body, improves symptoms and accelerates the body's natural healing power. After learning Reiki many students start to move into a more harmonious and balanced lifestyle. The body's natural communication mechanism starts to work again and one is more able to simply "know" what is good and what to avoid. On a personal note I stopped drinking coffee immediately after learning Reiki and have not drink coffee since.

- Mental - Reiki affects our deepest thoughts and conditioned ways of thinking, and leads to an open mind. Negative traits and patterns are reduced and a feeling of inner calm results.

- Emotional - Reiki flows deep into the subconscious mind and allows one to see the thought patterns that hold us back. Jealousy, anger, fear and other negative emotions start to be replaced by an unconditional love and understanding of life and its differences.

- Spiritual - After Reiki many students become much more loving, compassionate, and nonjudgmental and begin to understand that they are not separate in this universe, but part of a larger whole.

When we are in harmony with our thoughts and emotions, the body is also in harmony and we are at ease. All Dis-Ease is simply a moving away from this state of ease.

When this lack-of-ease happens the life force energy is disrupted and does not flow smoothly, thus leading to physical symptoms in the body.

HOW TO LEARN REIKI

Reiki is easy to use and you do not need any special equipment, just a pair of hands on your body! You can do it for yourself or others and it allows you to rebalance yourself on all 4 levels and to come back into a state of harmony.

Reiki is given by gently laying your hands on the clothed body of a person. Within seconds, the energy can be felt. The effects vary depending on the individual but may include a feeling of intense heat, tingling, swirling, coldness and even emotional outbursts.

Certain hand positions are taught corresponding to the physical organs and emotional states. For example the liver area associates with anger (it's interesting that we use the word livid to describe anger), the lungs with sadness, and the kidneys with fear or prejudice.

The chakras (energy centers of the body) are also balanced, as is the front and back torso, arms, legs and the head area.

When you are giving or receiving Reiki, the brain moves into alpha state, a state of deep relaxation. Both the giver and receiver connect with the energy and both benefit from the session. Reiki shows you the messages from your body and you start to see a new framework for language and ingrained behavior patterns.

Reiki truly is an amazing healing therapy and you sense the healing touch as soon as the Reiki hands are placed on the body.

Many believe that Reiki has its own intelligence and actually goes to the site of the problem in the body, regardless of where the hands are placed. I have seen numerous examples of this, one such example was when my hands were placed on the stomach area, and one of the legs of the client, where the problem exists, started to twitch.

Dr. Usui realized through his experience that receiving the healing energy alone is not enough to make a person whole and complete. The physical symptom is merely the fruit of the tree and so to bring about lasting change one needs to look at the roots of the problem. These are usually deep conditioned, subconscious, emotional issues.

He adopted the Meiji Emperor's principles for living life and incorporated them into Reiki therapy. There are 5 principles in total and all start with the words - 'Just for Today'.

This was done because Dr Usui realized if you can do something for just one day and then repeat it each day, you are more likely to succeed than if he said you had to change at once for your whole life.

Reiki in effect has 2 legs - the physical side of Reiki, with the laying on of hands, and the 5 principles which are about how you live life.

FOUR FORMS OF REIKI MEDITATION

Meditation is an integral part of Reiki, a traditional Japanese healing practice. According to the practitioners of Reiki, Reiki meditation can have a number of benefits, among them enhanced relaxation (leading to the healing of self), clairvoyance (ability to mystically foresee things), greater awareness and greater ability to visualize, which is important since we are more likely to achieve things we can visualize in life than things that we cannot visualize.

Reiki meditation is also the means to balance one's energy, which is what in Reiki parlance leads to the healing of oneself, and which is also what gives you the ability to heal others through Reiki via 'energy attunement'. Through Reiki meditation, one is also supposed to attain a sense of detachment, which would empower them to 'go with the flow' rather than trying to force things to happen, which is what one would be inclined to do in default; naturally leading to frustration throughout life as most things in life are things we cannot really control.

Reiki meditations can be seen as falling into four major forms.

First is breathing meditation, and this form of meditations is always a prelude to other forms. In one of the breathing forms of meditation, one is advised to breathe slowly, while focusing their thoughts on Reiki. In another form of breathing Reiki meditation, one is advised to breath 'naturally' (as opposed to breathing slowly), and this is usually employed towards the end of Reiki breathing meditation sessions, as one transitions from the meditative state to the 'ordinary' state, maybe in setting the stage for a Reiki healing session.

Another form of Reiki meditation is visualization-based meditation. Among the things visualized here include the Reiki symbol (for Reiki practitioners who have attained the second degree of Reiki training), as well as one's goals in which one is seeking Reiki's help in their attainment (since Reiki can also help in the attainment of ordinary day to day goals, beyond healing which is its most recognized application). The idea in the visualization-based Reiki meditation is to see the object of one's meditation with one's own 'third eye' - and doing so clearly.

Then there is postural meditation, where a Reiki practitioner is able to attain the meditative state through the use of various postures. This type of meditation is normally used as a prelude to the other types of meditations, including the breathing Reiki meditation (which is itself a prelude to things like Reiki visualization-meditation). In postural terms, meditation may be carried out while lying down or sitting, among other postures.

Another form of Reiki meditation is the moment to moment meditation, manifest through the way the practitioner goes about their day to day roles. This stems from the understanding that things like 'avoiding anger, avoiding worry, and devotion in one's vocation' are among the things required of a Reiki practitioner, on a moment to moment basis. And these also - combined with a detached attitude on a moment to moment basis can be termed as forms of meditation too.

REIKI MEDITATION TECHNIQUES

Focus and Tranquility

You practice meditation in order to find your inner peace and to regain your peaceful state both in mind and body. Through meditation one person can find harmony within itself and relax his mind. Having the necessary time to reflect and focus you find your energy balance.

A fundamental aspect to meditations is for you to create a focus point where to channel your energy. Your hands can act as a focus point for your energy. In this case you should keep your hands close to your chest in a prayer like formation. The middle fingers can help your mind stay in touch with your meditation by pressing the middle fingers together - they are a mean of refocusing.

Deep Thoughts and Deeper Breathing

In Reiki meditation the breathing techniques are more that essential if you want to reach an optima meditation session.

Through deep breathing you gain access to the spiritual body. Exhaling and inhaling thoroughly you can penetrate through different states of your body including mental and emotional body. You can ask a question or think of an idea while doing these exercises.

The idea or question can refer to anything from a person to a thing. You can keep your mind from straying from your purpose by using the fire fingers - the middle fingers. It's recommended that you should limit your meditation sessions to fifteen minutes when doing it the first time.

Emotions and Symbols

Using shorter meditation sessions allows you to find the best focusing and breathing methods. Only this way you'll have full control over your mind. You need this in order to stay focused through entire meditation. You need more than the power symbol if you want a full experience. You need to add to your meditation emotional and distance symbols. With these three symbols combined you can use the Reiki energy to heal you or others. At the same time you can use this energy to counter the effects of your negative feelings.

The more you practice the more comfortable you'll be through your meditation session and you'll have a better control over your mind and body. Deep breathing and the use of your hands help you channel the energy from your toes up to the head. You need to practice Reiki meditation for years in order to reach all the meditation levels.

The Reiki principles help us in turning the negative energy from our body to positive energy and that translates into a better state of being. Meditation can help us clear our mind and keep a healthier body.

5 WAYS TO USE REIKI

Apart from self-healing and treating others Reiki can be used for other applications. This is what makes Reiki different to other healing methods and alternative therapies as it can be used in many aspects of our daily lives.

Reiki can even be used on inanimate objects. So next time you have a problem with your computer or one of your plants is dying remember that here is one way you can use Reiki.

The fundamental reason for this is that Reiki is just a way of transferring energy to where there is an imbalance. Everything in the Universe is made from energy - even inanimate objects.

- Plants and flowers - life energy belongs as much to plants and flowers as it does to humans and animals, so the healing power of Reiki can be applied to them. For house plants put your hands around the pot to focus sending energy to the roots - this is where the plant draws its sustenance and where most effort should be focused. When you sense enough Reiki energy has been transferred then moves your hands to the upper part of the plant. For outdoor plants you should focus on the seeds / bulbs before you plant them as it is impossible to give Reiki to the whole garden unless you master Distance healing.

• Food and drink - we draw our energy from the food and drink we consume. It therefore makes sense to put into our stomachs not only good food but good energy. Give Reiki to food as it cooks or when it is on the table and fill it with good energy. Even foods that are bad for you can be improved - but not made good! With Reiki. If you don't believe this try taking a glass of tap water and taste it - then give the water Reiki and taste again.

- Animals - this isn't really any different to treating a human except you will have to be more intuitive and try to be guided by the animal. For fish you can place your hands in the tank, and for animals you can't / don't want to touch use distance healing.

- Your environment - this can be more advanced but all levels of Reiki practitioners can do this. Place your hands on the walls of a room and offer Reiki energy transference. If your house isn't selling this method can work as the environment becomes much nicer and has a better feel.

- Distance Healing - this isn't unique to Reiki but is generally carried out a little differently. You can send Reiki to people on the other side of the world. Whilst this sounds hard to believe it is done by using visualization, which brings the focus of the healing to the fore. Photographs are often used. You can also send Reiki into the future to support your actions. See yourself in the situation where you want the support and send Reiki to yourself.

THE BASICS OF REIKI TREATMENT

What is Reiki treatment?

If you have heard about Reiki but are not sure what it is, this is a great opportunity to learn the basics so you can make a wise decision.

Reiki is an ancient Japanese healing technique that uses and manipulates energy at different levels with the intention to heal, make well, mend and restore health. This is achieved through the balancing of the Chakras or energy centers located throughout the spine. When balance is achieved, the spirit, the mind, the emotions, and the body are in harmony.

It's been said that many spiritual healers of all times have used Reiki as a healing technique. The Reiki which the contemporary world is familiar with today is the same concept that was rediscovered by Mikao Usui in the earlier part of the 20th century. However, the strategies have been modified and adapted throughout time. The main techniques have been used by many Reiki Masters and according to their individual results; the techniques have been mixed and matched which explains the more than 40 modalities that we find nowadays.

The variations that exist are based on diverse interpretations and belief systems. The main point here is that all modalities of Reiki work, because they are all based in the same principle, that of utilizing energy to heal the individual. It is important to note that Reiki is not related in any way to religion or faith. It exists in its own consciousness of energy which is shared by all living creatures and human beings regardless of faith.

Understanding the Reiki Treatment

In order to achieve a clearer understanding of Reiki and its treatment technique, it is necessary to dig a bit deeper. First, we must study the foundation of illness and understand how and why it develops. Secondly, we must spend some time in reflection on the essence of health, well-being and life in general.

Generally speaking, allopathic medicine looks at the human body as a mechanical gadget, much like a clock with all of its elements. Thus, when one of its parts stops functioning, gets out of synch or becomes somehow damaged, it aims to restore, repair or replace the problem area.

One typical way of handling this human body dilemma is by prescribing drugs and performing surgeries. This is not to say that allopathic medicine doesn't have its rightful place in the healing practice. It is definitely helpful in many conditions, such as in the case of broken bones, acute infections or when the need for emergency intervention is vital to preserve life.

However, let's not forget that in many instances the human body can repair itself when it is given proper nutrition, time and overall attention and care. Thus, instead of running to the drug cabinet for some analgesic pill as soon as you have a headache, you may want to consider using Reiki to heal yourself.

Another example relates to chronic conditions for which allopathic medicine doesn't seem to have a clear answer yet. For instance, arthritis is one ailment for which some treatments provide temporary relief while some others are not effective at all. Worse yet, some medications may carry great risks to other organs and systems.

On the other hand, comprehensive or holistic medicine such as the Reiki modality employs a very different approach in addressing the human body and its functions. It is based on respect for the body's wisdom to heal itself as well as looking at the mental, emotional, physical, and spiritual components as a whole.

A holistic approach assumes that when one part of the body is malfunctioning, the rest of the body's structures get affected as well; so, in order to get to the root of the problem, the cause that has created disharmony must be tracked down. Signs and symptoms arise as a way for the body to indicate that something is out of balance. These warning signs shouldn't be ignored as they may lead to more serious health problems.

The Main Role of the Practitioner in the Reiki treatment

Reiki practitioners emphasize that warning signs should never be ignored no matter how insignificant they may seem. They may be an indication that something more serious is developing. Thus, Reiki practitioners address this concern by making use of the Reiki energy to release blockages and restructure the free flow of energy which can heal the problematic organs and tissues.

Once the symptoms are eliminated, they will encourage a change of lifestyle that may include revision of diet, rest and sleep, physical activity, personal affairs and stress, and even evaluation of the relationship between work, values and fulfillment. They will guide and instruct you on how to keep a balanced life for your overall well-being.

And this is why the Reiki treatment has been regarded as extremely valuable. From the time of its rediscovery, this healing technique has never faltered when practiced correctly. It is more needed than ever to live in balance and harmony in these troubled days of stress and concern. Reiki can and will help when you give yourself the opportunity to experience it.

And, most importantly, it won't hurt to give it a try. The side effect will only be a feeling of bliss.

The "Reiki Master Training" site is dedicated to those who want to explore and learn about this magnificent healing art, as well as for those who are interested in becoming a Reiki Master through distant learning.

USING A PENDULUM DURING REIKI HEALING TREATMENTS

Reiki Masters and practitioners can benefit from using pendulums during Reiki healing treatments in many ways. Below we will discuss the three most common ways to use a pendulum on clients during Reiki sessions. But remember; feel free to think outside of the box! Pendulums can help you gain wisdom beyond what your conscious mind knows if you let them.

1. Use your Reiki pendulum to determine the health of the seven main chakras of the client.

The chakras are energy centers in your body, and the word literally means 'wheel' in Sanskrit. The seven main chakras (the root, sacral chakra, solar plexus, heart, throat, third eye and crown) should all be spinning in a clockwise direction if they are healthy.

People's chakras can often become blocked with energy, or have too little or too much energy in them. Directing the healing Reiki energy specifically toward these imbalanced chakras is an excellent way to return them to their balanced state. If you hold your Reiki pendulum over each chakra at the very beginning of your session, you can determine which chakras need extra attention and plan your Reiki healing treatment accordingly.

Be sure to check the chakras at the end of the Reiki session as well! It is always nice to see the progress and how the Reiki healing energy has helped the client.

2. Let the pendulum tell you what to do during the Reiki treatment (i.e. where to stand, which symbols to give)

In order to use your pendulum effectively, you need to determine how its responses before the Reiki treatment. For example, you will already want to know how your pendulum replies 'Yes', 'No', 'Maybe', 'I don't know' and 'Ask later' before you start your Reiki session. You can determine your pendulum's responses by programming and understanding your Reiki pendulum beforehand.

Assuming you have already programmed your Reiki pendulum and understand its answers, use it as the valuable tool it is during your Reiki treatments and ask it questions about anything which you are uncertain. You may be at your client's feet, and ask your pendulum if you should remain at the foot of the table or move to the person's head. Also, a great question to 'ask' is which symbols to use during the Reiki healing. Instead of asking questions, say statements for a better response from your Reiki pendulum. For example, say, "I should use the forgiveness symbol over the client's heart," and wait to see your Reiki pendulum's response. Once again, use your creativity!

3. Determine when to give Reiki treatments and which complementary modalities to use during the session

Many Reiki practitioners incorporate the use of crystals; sound healing, aromatherapy, acupressure and energy work into their Reiki treatment sessions. Let your pendulum help you determine not only which complementary tools to use, but also when to schedule the sessions to get the most out of them.

While using a Reiki pendulum can be an invaluable tool during your treatments, the beauty of the Reiki healing energy is that it has intelligence in and of itself. So essentially, there is no wrong way to use your pendulum. Even if you think you are making a 'mistake' - which is really just an opportunity to learn- the Reiki healing energy will always travel to where it is needed most. So have fun with your Reiki pendulum!

CHAPTER 6
SYMBOLS IN REIKI

Symbols are pictorial triggers that are commonly used in meditation as a point of focus or as a tool for visualization in order to achieve a higher sense of awareness and energy manifestation. A symbol aims at the psyche and the subconscious mind to condense the meaning of a whole philosophy into a single symbol.

This same principle is used in Reiki to aid meditation, healing and evoking positive Reiki energy. But it is important to remember that the symbol in itself is not a source of power but the healing treatment and Reiki energy comes from the healer.

Reiki symbols are generally kept secret till the initiate reaches the second level. The symbols for Reiki are based loosely on the Japanese system of writing, Kanji. They are generally taught during the Reiki level 2 - Attunement. However each person is unique and the subconscious of each attunes to these symbols in a different manner based to various factors like intent and psychic energies so it may happen that you may come across variations of these symbols with different Masters. There is no fixed rule for drawing these and therefore nobody is actually wrong.

There are many misunderstandings concerning these symbols, one of which is that they are supposed to draw the symbols in a particular order. These symbols are generally derived from Japanese writing where the style of writing the characters is different from the western world and the writing is done with emphasis on style, direction and order but this is only done for legibility purposes and bears no relevance to the meaning of the symbol or its power in Reiki. Though the Reiki symbols are each used for a specific purpose there are some who prefer to use these symbols combined during Reiki treatments in order to boost the power of the Reiki. This is generally done to make a Reiki healing more effective.

HOW TO MAKE REIKI POWER SYMBOLS WORK FOR YOU!

A reiki course is quite simple in principle: via a simple course of treatment, a student is initiated into the use of reiki energies via a series of ever more precise and powerful 'attunements', which contain a fantastically powerful form manipulating reiki energies effectively. These attunements also have a massively powerful effect on the body, containing and aligning the forces and energies that course through it.

The differing rates at which these energies spin necessitates the partition of reiki courses into three separate levels, according the normal reiki teaching method. In the final stage of reiki instruction, the stage at which the student of reiki finally achieves mastery and the right to use these energies for their personal good and for the good of others, certain reiki power symbols are taught to them by their master. These will be discussed below.

Nowadays, it has become possible, thanks to the Internet and to the explosion of reiki courses throughout the world, to attain the first two levels of reiki mastery within a matter of days. This leads to a stronger reiki attunement, in the experience of respected reiki practitioners. The final control over reiki is signified and carried out by use of the reiki power symbol, which we shall discuss below.

The reiki master attunes the student by acting as a conduit, using his or her hands to alter the energy flows of the student, thereby creating a conduit which allows the energy to flow through the both of them unimpeded.

The cosmic energy that reiki practitioners use is thereby given free play in the body, and the flows from the base of the spine to the top of their head. This river of pure energy is the secret behind the efficacy of reiki energy and the popularity of reiki as a healing method - frequently, both reiki practitioners and patients feel refreshed after a session. This makes these attunements a special experience for both parties, another benefit of reiki.

Stage one of the attunement process, which is meant to benefit the physical, corporeal self of the student, is not where reiki symbols are taught. That comes later, during the second stage, wherein the student is taught the uses of these power symbols as well as the importance of using the right ones for their ends and needs. This attunement opens up the body and allows it access to the spiritual energy contained in the body of the master. The second stage, attunement level 2, is where the reiki symbols are introduced, along with the basic reiki symbol, the reiki power symbol.

Whereas the first stage is intended for the opening up of the energies of the body, the second stage sets the body's energies into motion and gives the student the power to contain them and use them beneficially. So the use of the reiki power symbol lies in stage 2, alongside the distance symbol, and the mental symbol. The power symbol is the basic symbol of the reiki method, as it is what signifies the power of the student over the energies that course through his or her body.

CHAPTER 7
REIKI STONES

What are Reiki Stones?

Reiki, specifically, is the system of healing that believes, in using conduits, powerful, precise intra-universal life force energy may be utilized to create healing effects. This energy is commonly referred to as prana, mana, chi, source, and Holy Spirit.

This energy helps to promote healing effects in all types of living things on the material realm, as well as the mental, spiritual, and emotional levels. This energy may be utilized to heal nearly any type of ailment with nothing more than the sheer force of universal energy. In using this energy, all the true organic medicine may be better achieved without the use of even the most natural products.

More specifically, Reiki uses Ki, which is natural life force, to heal. This uses non-physical life force to alter the life force of an individual to create healing in some fashion. Using Reiki allows for the body, mind, and spirit to be healed simultaneously.

How does Reiki work?

Reiki may be used for everything that needs healing in some capacity. Some healers even are able to heal ailments that have not yet presented themselves yet, or emotion issues that lie in a person's past. It all depends on the ability of the healer and his or her understanding of the art of Reiki. It has been known to heal serious and life-threatening problems such as the flu, heart disease, sclerosis, and even cancer, but it also is able to heal minor problems such as colds, cuts, scrapes, broken bones, headaches, sunburns, insomnia, fatigue, sore throats, poor memory, impotence and even the lack of confidence.

The treatment basically fells like a warm light passing through your body, as it progresses, cold areas of the body are warmed. Those cold areas represent different ailments in the body that need healing. Thus, Reiki may be used to forgo negative side effects of western medicine, shorten healing time and eliminate pain.

Reiki utilizes Reiki healing stones that have individualized markings cut into them. These marking represent a specific type or style of healing for an individual healer. These stones act as a conduit from raw spiritual energy to the body. It cleanses the aura in the body by clearing out negative energy in the chakras. It also helps diminish doubtful or untrue thoughts about oneself to better achieve spiritual awareness. In clearing out the negativity, the body is able to better function and extract negative materials with the new energy granted by the healer.

Just by clearing out the chakras, the raw energy is able to heal even the most severe ailment. In this way, Reiki may be used on any person of any religion, or any plane of spiritual thought. All people have these chakras, thus, all people may be susceptible to the healing power of a Reiki stone and a Reiki healer. Reiki's healing power is more than just the reliving of symptoms, it is the actual, true healing of the potent negative energy that corrupts the body and effectively kills a certain part of the spirit by clogging the chakras. All that Reiki truly does is free the chakras so that the body is whole.

Reiki is an ancient art that has been used for several thousand years. With its healing power, most any ailment, large and small, may be fully healed to the core.

ALL ABOUT CRYSTAL HEALING REIKI

Reiki treatment is considered a form of spiritual energy healing, which is believed to be guided by the vast intelligence of the universe, or Universal Life Force, that which we have come to know as the mind of God.

Crystal Healing Reiki is widely used by many Reiki healers. Their use aids in the balancing of energy within the body which in turn helps in the therapeutic process. Reiki practitioners use crystals because they can speed up the healing.

The purpose behind laying crystals or gemstones is basically to aid in the releasing of physical, emotional, spiritual or mental blocks. It is believed that negative experiences, both physical and emotional, can cause blocks in the energy paths which in turn bring about disease.

The gemstones are laid on specific points of the body where the chakras or energy centers are located. The practitioner's role is to be comforting, non-judgmental, and supportive making the patient feel "safe" in case he feels the need to release his emotions verbally. In many instances, the healing begins once the patient feels the freedom to express himself. This is an integral part of the healing process.

Reiki healers seem to have a preference for quartz, since it is a clear and harmonically shaped crystal, which properties apparently clear the blockages within the body. However, since chakras are associated with colors according to the energy fields they represent, many practitioners will take this into consideration when choosing the crystals to be used during treatment.

It is believed that these crystals have unique vibrational energies connected to their color and shape. This seems to help in the balancing, realigning and amplifying of energy fields within the body. It is important to always use a stone that feels good to the patient when placed on his body. If any discomfort is felt, the crystal should be removed at once. A variety of stones can be used and interchanged during treatment, and once the patient has 'absorbed' the energy from one stone, it should be removed. For this to be effective, the practitioner and the client must work closely together during this process.

The gemstones should be cleaned and kept in optimal conditions so they keep their energetic properties. Thus, after treatment the gems should be placed in salt water, and some Masters recharge them through specific techniques.

The following are some of the crystals used for Crystal Healing Reiki:

- For the pelvic area, onyx, garnet and ruby can be used. The colors that represent these chakras are brown, black and red.

- For the abdominal area, tiger's eye, quartz and amber are used. The color associated to this area is gold.

- For the Third Eye or forehead, moss agate, amethyst and sodalite are indicated. The colors of this area are dark blue and purple.

- For the throat area, turquoise, aquamarine and amazonite are indicated. The colors associated with this area are light blue or blue green.

- For the crown or top of the head, quartz is used. The color of this stone is clear white.

- For the heart area, pink tourmaline, rose quartz, rhodonite, aventurine, and green tourmaline can be used. And the colors associated are pink and green.

- For the solar plexus, stones like malachite, peridot, rhodochrosite and moonstone can be used. The colors of this area are coral and chartreuse.